Grandma's Frugal Meals

Easy tips, techniques and old-time dishes

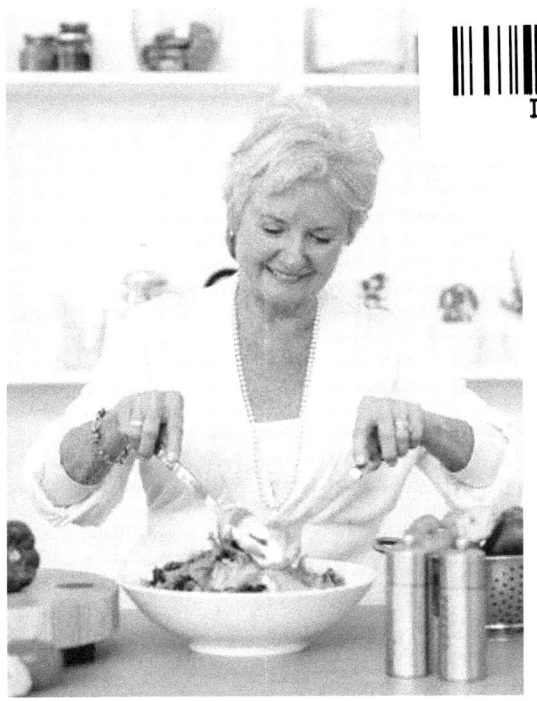

Dueep J. Singh

Mendon Cottage Books

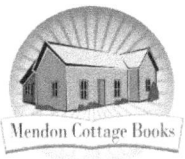

JD-Biz Publishing

All Rights Reserved.

No part of this publication may be reproduced in any form or by any means, including scanning, photocopying, or otherwise without prior written permission from JD-Biz Corp Copyright © 2014

All Images Licensed by Fotolia and 123RF.

Disclaimer

The information is this book is provided for informational purposes only. It is not intended to be used and medical advice or a substitute for proper medical treatment by a qualified health care provider. The information is believed to be accurate as presented based on research by the author.

The contents have not been evaluated by the U.S. Food and Drug Administration or any other Government or Health Organization and the contents in this book are not to be used to treat cure or prevent disease.

The author or publisher is not responsible for the use or safety of any diet, procedure or treatment mentioned in this book. The author or publisher is not responsible for errors or omissions that may exist.

Warning

The Book is for informational purposes only and before taking on any diet, treatment or medical procedure, it is recommended to consult with your primary health care provider.

Our books are available at

1. Amazon.com
2. Barnes and Noble
3. Itunes
4. Kobo
5. Smashwords
6. Google Play Books

All Rights Reserved.

No part of this publication may be reproduced in any form or by any means, including scanning, photocopying, or otherwise without prior written permission from JD-Biz Corp Copyright © 2014

All Images Licensed by Fotolia and 123RF.

Disclaimer

The information is this book is provided for informational purposes only. It is not intended to be used and medical advice or a substitute for proper medical treatment by a qualified health care provider. The information is believed to be accurate as presented based on research by the author.

The contents have not been evaluated by the U.S. Food and Drug Administration or any other Government or Health Organization and the contents in this book are not to be used to treat cure or prevent disease.

The author or publisher is not responsible for the use or safety of any diet, procedure or treatment mentioned in this book. The author or publisher is not responsible for errors or omissions that may exist.

Warning

The Book is for informational purposes only and before taking on any diet, treatment or medical procedure, it is recommended to consult with your primary health care provider.

Check out some of the other Healthy Gardening Series books at Amazon.com

Gardening Series on Amazon

Check out some of the other Health Learning Series books at Amazon.com

Health Learning Series on Amazon

Table of Contents

Introduction

Knowing what to cook was as important as knowing how to cook, for grandma. She also learned how to make the best of whatever was in front of her, from her grandmother, and so on for centuries. Millenniums ago, her ancestors when gathering in the woods for herbs and vegetables while the menfolk of the family trapped and hunted for meat, game and anything else edible and delicious.

It was then grandma's many times great-grandmother's job to make all these ingredients into something delicious and healthy as well as palatable and nourishing. So she used her instinct and her creativity to make delicacies with the ingredients available at hand.

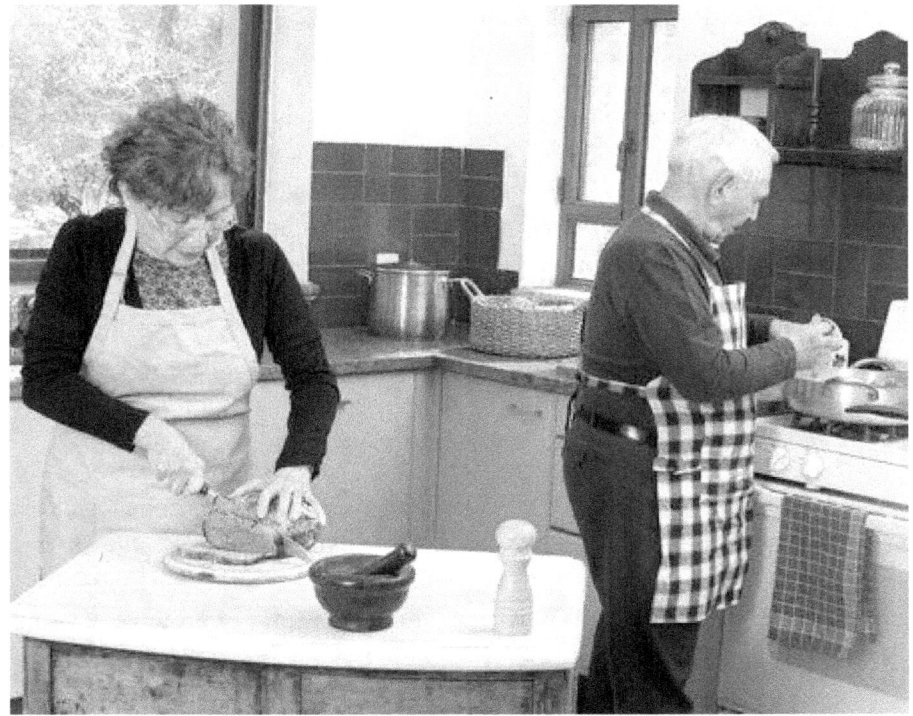

Although science-fiction already has stories about scientists making complete little nutritional packages in the shape of pills that are going to take the shape of food in the coming centuries, we are very fortunate that we do not have to face that sort of blandness in our meals today.

We still have the good fortune of going to the nearest market or the nearest organic garden and collecting fresh greens, as well as herbs. We have plenty of fresh meat at hand. And best of all, we have all the ingredients to make good wholesome food.

We only hope, judging by the pleasure most of us get from eating, the preparation, cooking and serving of this nutritious food is going to be a human activity which is going to be around for a long time.

But most of us cannot afford to have some of the more exotic ingredients, of which we dream. Either they are not available to us in our city. Or perhaps they are beyond our budget. Unfortunately, for a large percentage of people all over the world, budget constraints are the reason why they have to make do with makeshift meals instead of eating what nature intended for them – good wholesome, natural ingredients.

Grandma was a frugal person. She lived in a time when the dollars earned by grandpa had to be stretched in such a manner that the whole family could be fed and fed well. Times changed and times of prosperity came along, and the eating habits of the whole family changed. Instead of two or three healthy meals in a day, there was food aplenty and the whole family could now afford to eat whatever they wanted, whenever they wanted, and in large quantities.

This naturally gave rise to problems including obesity. Also, by not regulating the meal intake as well as the quality of the meals, the quality of the general health of grandma's children deteriorated as time went by.

However, the circle of financial constraints has gone and come around again and the time for tightening belts and looking at our budgets has become the top priority. A majority of us all over the world again are looking for ways and means in which we can get the proper nutrition in the form of proteins, vitamins, minerals and energy, which our bodies required to keep functioning in a healthy manner.

Grandma's Tips for Food Substitutions

High-protein Food items like eggs, fish, meat and poultry are affordable items, which are a part of one's diet. One serving a day of any of these items is enough. Have an egg for breakfast. Make sure that liver is a part of your meals, because of its exceptionally high vitamin and iron values.

If you are a vegetarian, you can substitute dried beans and cheese for meat. While cooking meals, you can substitute nonfat dry milk in recipes or mix with whole milk. Not only is it very good and economical but is also lower in cholesterol.

Use plain yogurt in place of sour cream for dips and on potatoes. You can make your own yogurt very inexpensively using nonfat dry milk, regular milk and yogurt culture.

How to Make Perfect Yogurt

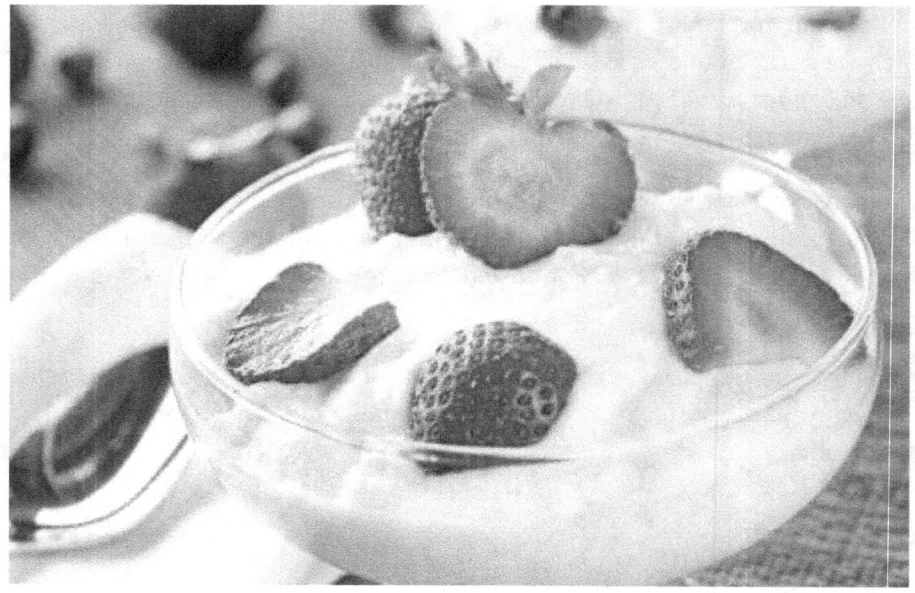

Yogurt was one very healthy dish, along with the buttermilk and butter made fresh from the collected cow's milk of the day, made by grandma if she had a cow. The traditional way of making yoghurt is made by boiling the milk and then cooling it down to room temperature. If you get pasteurized milk, boil it to room heat.

Milk was always boiled before drinking, traditionally in the East, to get rid of germs and also foreign particles. It was then strained. Even now, pasteurized milk is still boiled, even though it has already been boiled and packaged. That is because the majority of people in the East do not trust the pasteurizing process and would rather boil it again before use, than drink it straight from the milk bottle or from the packet.

So boil 1 L of milk. Allow to cool until it is lukewarm. You are going to see a thin layer of cream floating on top. You can keep it to add some taste you are making yogurt.

You need 3 tablespoons full of yogurt culture.

What Is Yogurt Culture?

It is just the remainder of the yogurt, which was left behind after you finished the yogurt you made yesterday. Remember to keep at least 2 to 3 tablespoons full and do not empty out that yogurt bowl.

Dip your finger in the milk. If it is tolerably warm, in the warm weather, this is the time you put in the yogurt. Whip it briskly with a spoon, cover with a lid, and placed by one side of the stove in your warm kitchen. This is normally made overnight, so that you have perfect yogurt to eat for breakfast the next morning. The next morning, it has set, so put it in the fridge.

Also, I found a friend setting yogurt in cold weather, – freezing Missouri weather – by warming up her oven at 125°C for five minutes. Then she put in the yogurt container in the oven and left it overnight. Good idea!

If you really want a traditional exotic flavor and taste, boil this milk in a red earthernware pot, allow it to cool to lukewarm, add the culture, and leave the yogurt to set. This is considered to be one of the most delicious ways in which to eat milk products and meat products in many parts of the East – cooking in earthenware pots.

This yogurt is going to have the taste of mother Earth, in a sweetened form.[I still cannot understand how that yogurt got sweet. I never added any sugar to it.] It is also going to have a distinctly delicious wet earthenware aroma, which many gourmets consider fascinating.

This yogurt is excellent for eating on its own, as a dip, or as an accompaniment. You can also use it as a marinade for meat. Churn it to make butter and buttermilk.

Meat

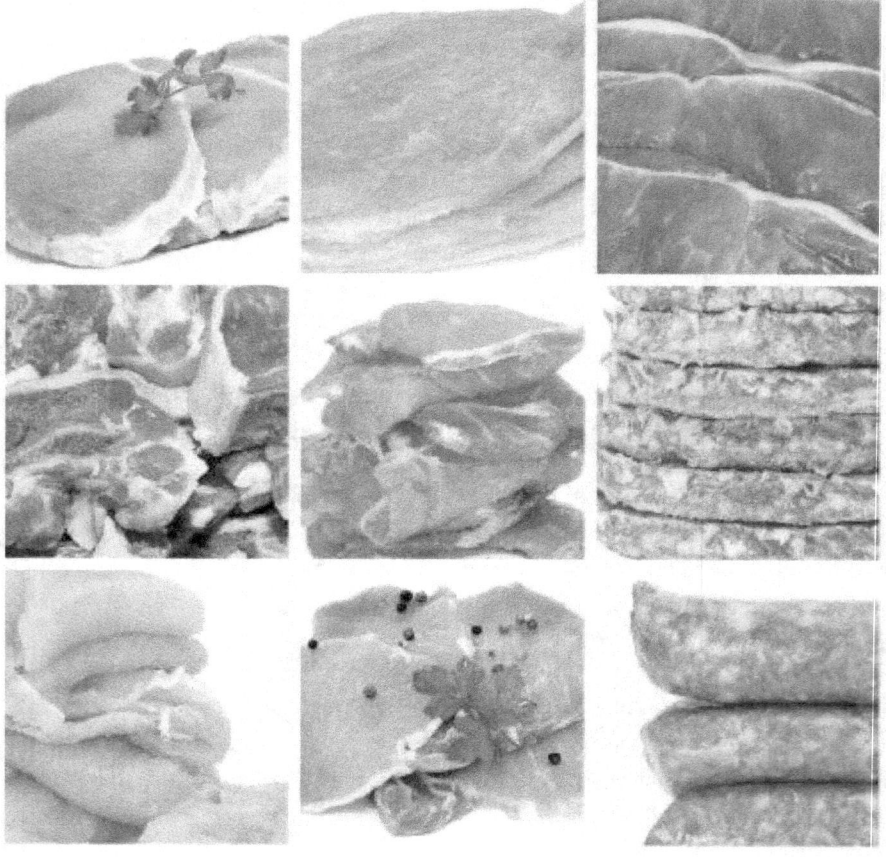

Meat is going to include red meat, white meat, game, poultry, venison, beef, pork, and any other animal products, either available to you fresh from the farm or, as is so common now, packaged. Meat uses up most of our budget dollars and that is why the cost can be shaved considerably if you buy meat whole and cut it up yourself. Whole chicken is cheaper than packaged buying fryers.

Also, let me tell you one secret about these fryers found on meat trays at the butchers. I know a person who has a poultry farm. One day I happened to go there, when birds were being prepared for the market. I noticed that the pullets and the fryers were dressed and then they were plumped into a barrel full of water.

I thought that the poultry farmer was being rather conscientious, cleaning the birds for the market, before sending them. It was only later, that I found that those fryers *absorbed the water* and the bird which went to the market and was being sold for around 800 g was just around 650 g. This is, of course, cheating of a high order, but then it happens all over the world.

So you need to be the butcher. You are going to save money, which would normally have been expended in paying the butcher to cut up the meat for you.

Hamburger is better priced in quantities over 5 pounds, so take it home and divided yourself into various portions. You can now make individual patties, meatloaf, or you can make servings of 1 pound. Spend a whole Sunday, making up different package for your freezer.

The best way to get meat is either to buy it in bulk from a trustworthy butcher, or buy it from a meatpacking house or farm, if you have one nearby. Buying meat from a reliable butcher means that you have done a little bit of comparison shopping on the prices and the quality, and the butcher is going to keep you on what is a good price buy or what is especially nice that week.

If you or any other family member is so inclined, you can catch your main course. If there is more than you can eat, freeze it. If you are a hunter, you can vary the menu according to the season by getting rabbit, grouse and squirrel. Yes, squirrel is tasty, if prepared properly. So you are going to save on food bills, if you enjoy hunting.

Choosing the right meat To Buy

Practically all of the meat sold in markets today should be inspected, either by federal or provincial meat inspectors. Nevertheless, there are many parts of the world where the meat goes straight from the farm to the consumer's table. So if you are living in an area where the meat is inspected regularly, make sure that the inspected stamp guarantees that the meat is from healthy animals than that the packing plants and the slaughter houses have met rigid sanitation standards.

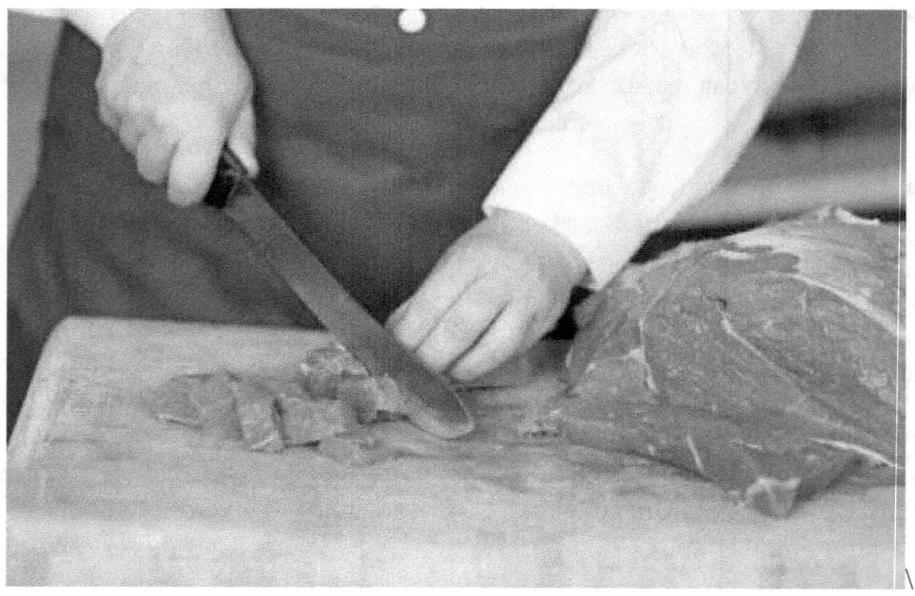

Inspected meat may be graded according to fat content. Some already inspected meat may be graded to a lower grade, even though it is healthy and wholesome. This is sometimes sold at a lower price. So if you can get it, why not.

Prices are going to vary, according to the cuts and according to the supply and demand. As a rule, the less tender cuts are going to be lower in price. These are at their best, when you cook them on moist heat – stewed, braised or pot roasted.

The more tender cuts are best, when you cook them with dry heat – broiled, oven roasted, or pan broiled.

Storing Meat

Consider the cost in terms of cost per serving, not the price per pound.

Cuts	Yield per Pound
Boneless, and trimmed of excess fat	Four servings
Small amount of bone and trimmed	Three – Four Servings
Medium amount of bone, some excess fat	two – three servings
Large amount of bone with gristle and excess fat	one – two servings.

The fresh meat should be unwrapped as soon as possible after purchase. Place it on a plate and cover loosely with waxed paper or transparent wrap. Store in a refrigerator and use within three or four days. Use ground meat within one – two days.

Smoked and cured meats may be left in their original wrappings, refrigerated and used within a week.

Frozen meat should be put in your freezer immediately in their packing and kept frozen until you are ready to cook it. Most fresh meats will keep for several months at 0°F or lower.

Baked Meat Patties

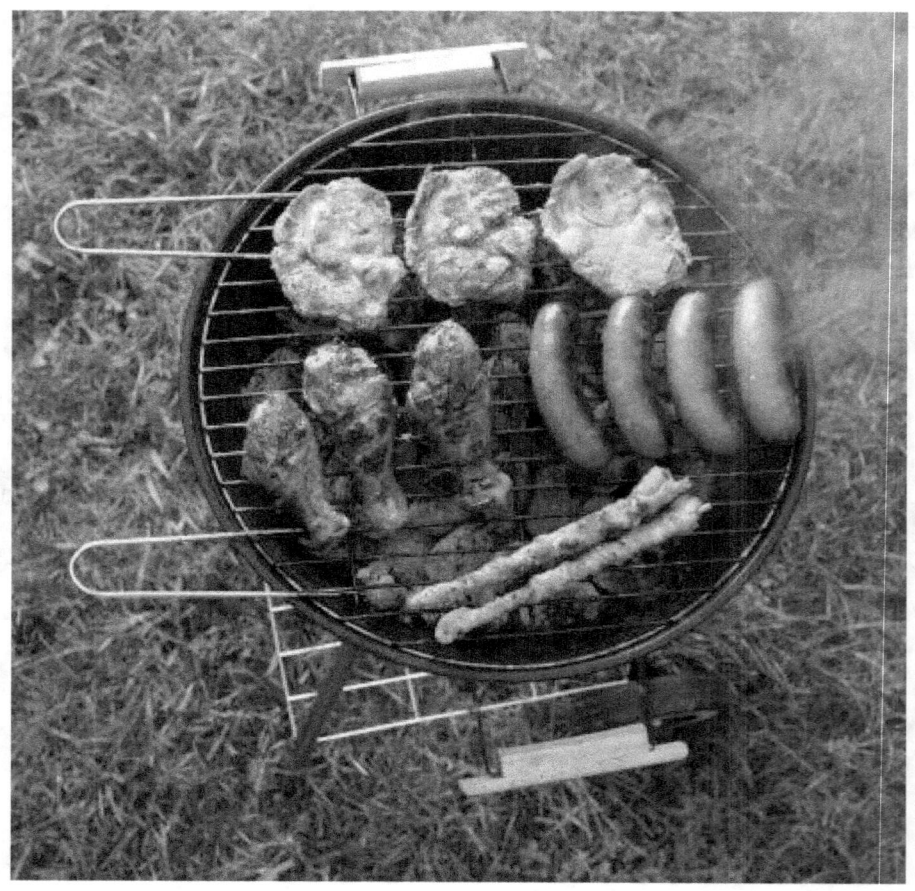

You can also make meat patties by grinding up the Chuck meat and frying it on a griddle. Excellent for hamburger and hot dog fillings.

1 ½ pounds ground beef or veal.
Half cup soft breadcrumbs or quick cooking rolled oats
2 tablespoons salt
Half teaspoon pepper
Half teaspoon dried mustard
One medium onion chopped
Half a cup vegetable stock, or milk or tomato juice.
Combine the meat, seasoning, crumbs and onions. Mix with the liquid.

Shape lightly into six patties and placed on a greased shallow baking pan. Bake in moderate oven, for 350°F for forty-five minutes. Serves six.

Meat patty Variations

1. You can wrap up each patty in a strip of bacon. Secure with a toothpick and bake as above.

2. Spread a layer of meat mixture in a pan, then a layer of bread crumbs, then another layer of meat mixture and possibly mashed potatoes. Add any herbs you like. Cover with another layer of meat mixture and bake about one hour.

3. Spread a layer of meat mixture into greased loaf pan. Arrange a row of hard cooked eggs end to end down the center. Cover with the remaining meat mixture. Bake for an hour.

How to Cure Your Own Hams

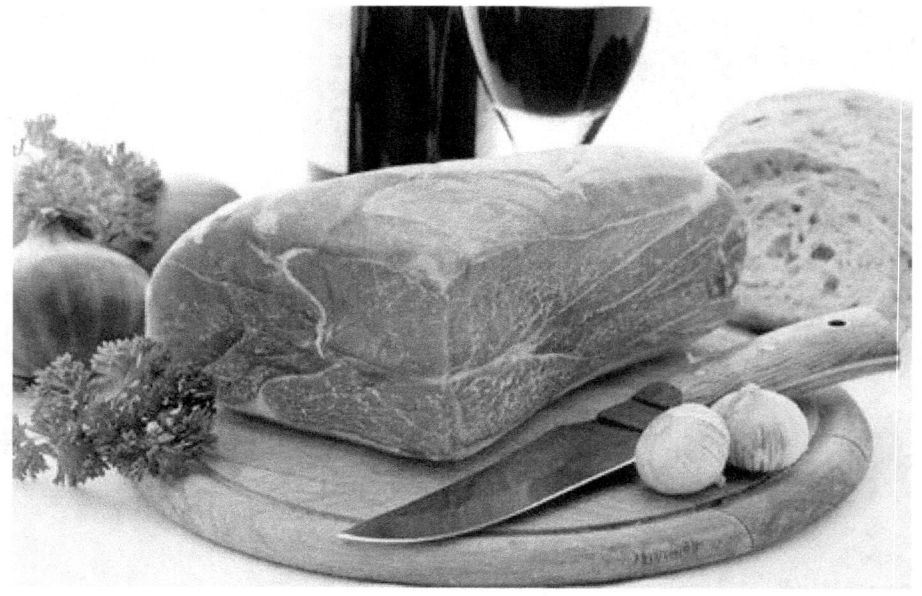

You can get nearly deli- level quality of cured hams by using traditional curing methods, especially the one given below.

This traditional way of curing your own hams is still a well-known secret in those mountains fastnesses where moonshine, Mountain Dew, white Lightnin' and other homemade brews are still a part of a lifestyle, one step ahead of the revenuer.

You can cure eight hams with this recipe.

Rub each ham well, with a mixture of 8 quarts of salt, 16 tablespoons of black pepper, and 16 tablespoons of white sugar. Put some mixture into the shank bone. Wrap up in brown paper and place in cloth bag. Hang in your cellar with shank down.

This URL is also very informative about choosing the best meat when you are making a ham.

http://schmidling.com/ham.htm

I liked it, especially when I have been using brine and spices to cure and make hams for quite a long while. I thought my method, learned from a farmer was his family secret, until I found out that East or West, the basics and procedures for preserving and curing meats down the ages have remained basically the same!

The cure that I have given you is going to give your ham more flavor and the extra last touch of je ne sais quoi de la piquante.

Other Food Found Outdoors

If you enjoy the outdoors, you can hunt for other things, which you can eat there. There are various berries, Hickory nuts, dandelion greens, watercress, rhubarb, Sassafras, and other wild edibles to be picked. Careful here – unless you really know what you are picking or go with somebody else who has the experience and knows his plants, do not pick up greens indiscriminately. Some are edible and some are not.

Here are two ways in which you can preserve rhubarb and Sassafras, which you collected during these rambles – by making them into jellies.

Rhubarb Jelly

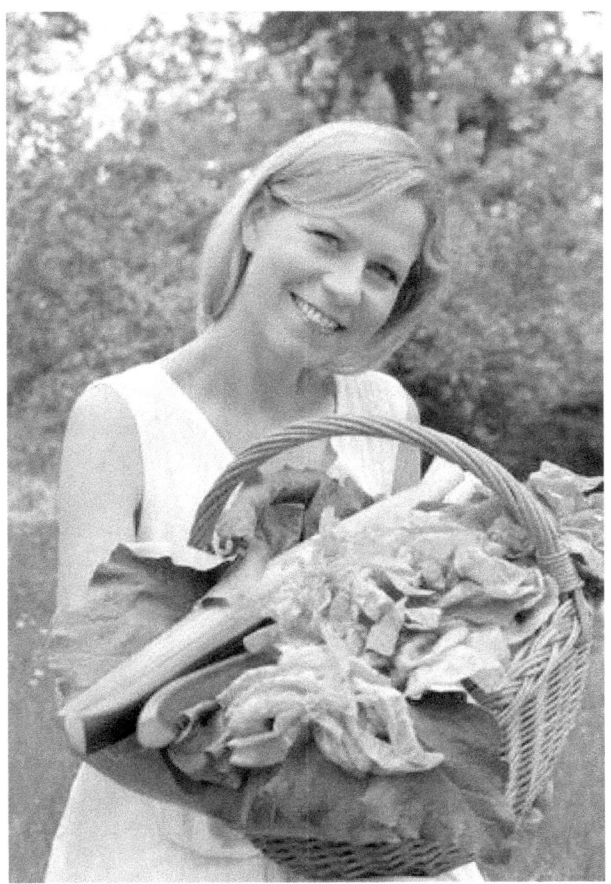

Never eat rhubarb leaves.

Rhubarb is a vegetable belonging to the same family as Sorrel. The stalks are thick and fleshy and have a tart flavor, that is why they work so well with sugar. **Never eat it raw.**

The leaves have poisonous oxalic acid, so make sure that you never eat them. Rhubarb leaves should be cut off and discarded. If the plant has a tough rib, cut it off with a sharp knife, after you have washed it. Now the stalk is ready for slicing and dicing, as thick or thin as you wish. You do not need to peel tender stalks of rhubarb. You just trim the bottom and the top of those stalks and slice them.

If you do not intend to eat them right now, you can store them in the fridge, by keeping their leaves on. But eat within the next two or three days.

To make a jelly you need –

Rhubarb – any quantity. 2 teaspoons granulated pectin, 1 cup honey

Wash and cut the rhubarb into 1 inch lengths. Place in preserving utensil. Grandma used a kettle. Add enough of water to prevent from sticking. Cook slowly in covered kettle until soft. Strain through a muslin bag.

Now, measure 1 cup juice, add 2 teaspoons granulated pectin and stir vigorously. Bring to boil, add 1 cup honey and continue to boil until jelly test is secured. This jelly test is done by putting a spoonful of jelly on a plate and pricking its surface with your finger. If the fruit "crinkles", it is done. It should solidify on the plate, when it comes in contact with the fresh air of your kitchen.

Fill hot and sterilized glasses with the jelly and cover with melted paraffin.

Sassafras Jelly

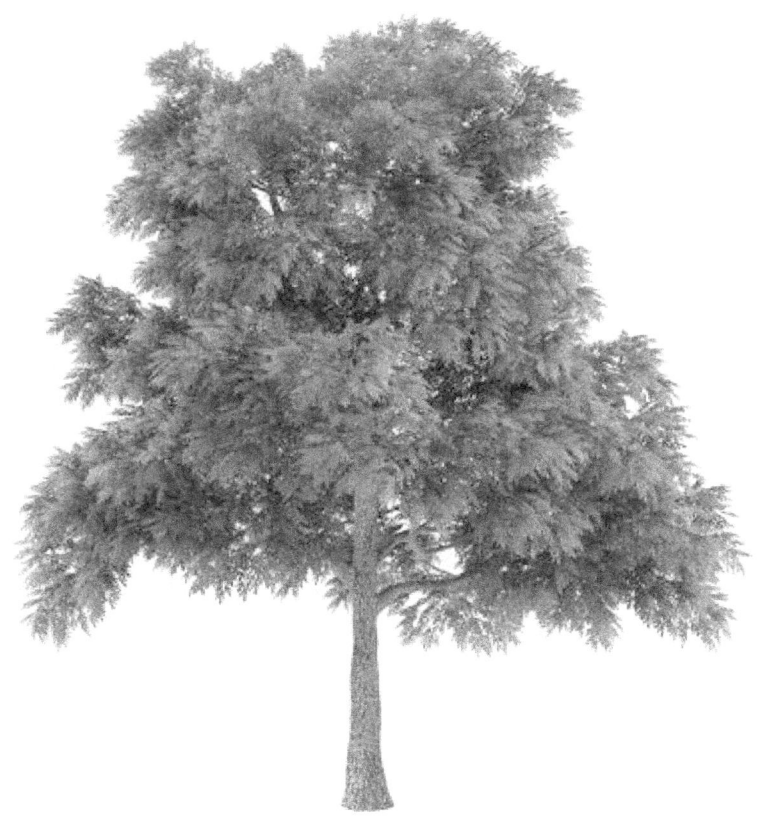

The dried leaves of the Sassafras tree are normally ground and used as a spice. Native Americans used Sassafras oil, bark and root extracts as an antiseptic and analgesic medicine to treat tooth aches, skin cures, dysentery, bronchitis, and even scurvy. This was a major export in the seventeenth century to Europe, especially because the wood was a highly prized item for making furniture.

If you find yourself in a wood, and need to start a fire, use Sassafras leaves and wood as a base. It is excellent flammable material because of its essential oils.

We are going to use Sassafras roots to make Sassafras jelly. Collect enough of roots to make 2 cups of a Tea, after it has been boil for half an hour and strained.

Now, measure out these 2 cups of Sassafras root tea, add a package of powdered pectin and just barely bring to a boil.

Add 3 cups of honey, [grandma used honey, because it was easier to obtain instead of sugar and healthier too…]. Now add 2 tablespoons full of Sassafras root bark which you have grated to a fine powder. Allow to simmer for six minutes. Put in sterilized glasses and covered with melted paraffin.

Dandelion Greens

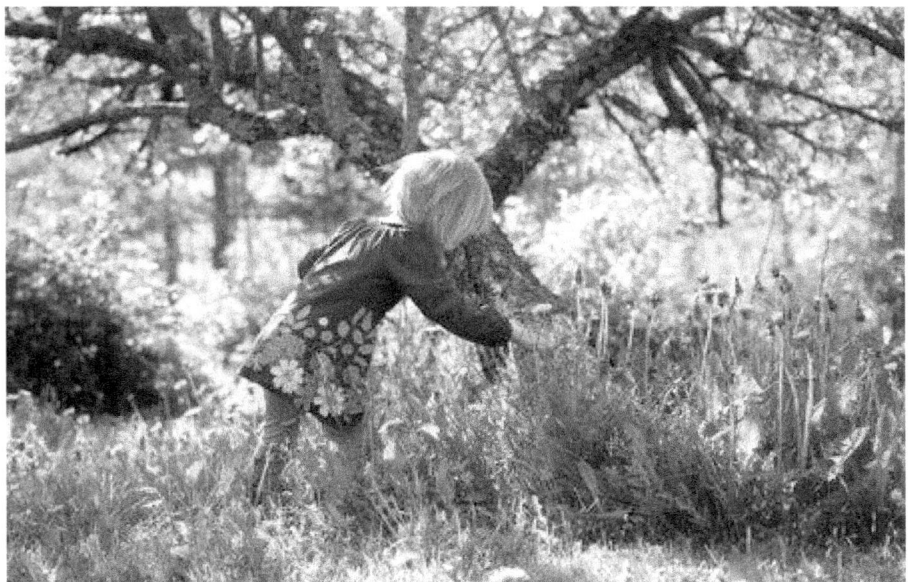

Good to look at, good to eat

Dandelions are really dandy eating as delicious herbs, which have been eaten as side dishes or as salad dishes down the centuries, accompanied with meat.

Dandelions can be used until they bloom. Every part of this plant can be eaten, roots, stems, leaves, etc. I have never heard of anybody eating them raw, – even though dandelion leaves, fresh picked are delicious to chomp upon like Nasturtium leaves – but I have tasted the leaves cooked with bacon. Delicious.

Anyway, pick these plants carefully, wash in several waters. Do not pick them, by the roadside, because the content of chemical pollutants, next to a road is considerably higher than when you pick them right in the woods. Put in boiling water with a piece of salt pork. Boil for one hour. [You can use bacon, like my friend Dianna did before she fed dandelion greens to me, and she said she did not have salt pork around. But the combination of both meat and greens is delicious.]

Drain well. Now add salted boiling water and boil for two more hours. When well done, and tender, drain and serve.

Luncheon Corn

Corn, especially on the cob is healthy and nutritious. But you can also use fresh corn to make baked dishes and really easily.

Cook **1 cup of broken macaroni** in salted boiling water. Drain and rinse in cold water. Place in baking dish. Beat **one egg, 1 cup milk, 1 cup corn, one teaspoonful salt, two teaspoonful sugar.** Pour over macaroni and dot with butter.

Bake in oven, 325 – 350°F for about twenty minutes. Garnish with parsley or watercress. You may grate cheese over the dish before baking, for added flavor.

Making Traditional Cornpone

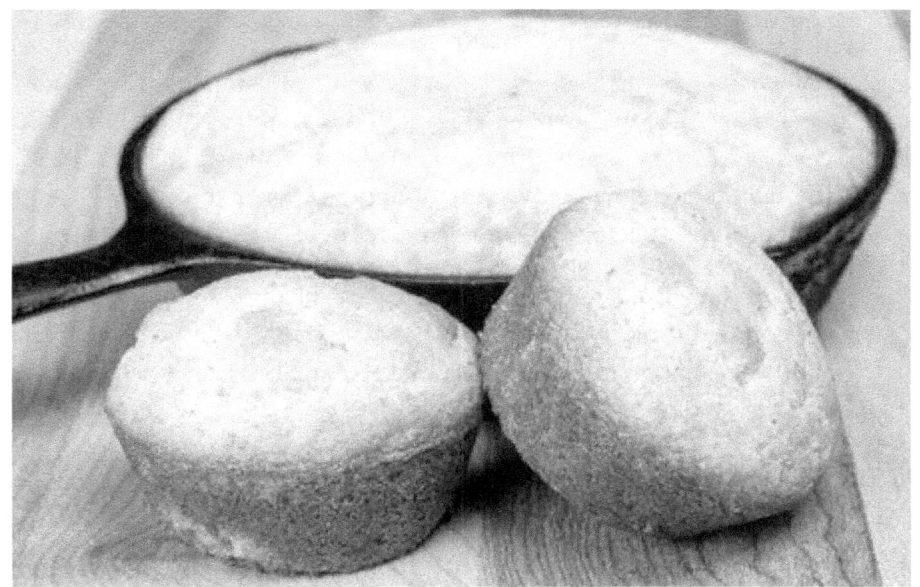

Apart from making Cornpone, you can also make cornmeal muffins.

While reading Kipling's story – *Brothers Square- Toes in Rewards and Fairies*,[1] I was struck by a gesture made by an Indian chief, when he met Gen. Washington.

That was a statelified meeting to behold—three big men, and two of 'em looking like jewelled images among the spattle of gay-coloured leaves. I saw my chiefs' war-bonnets sinking together, down and down. Then they made the sign which no Indian makes outside of the Medicine Lodges—a sweep of the right hand just clear of the dust and an inbend of the left knee at the same time, and those proud eagle feathers almost touched his boot-top.'

'What did it mean?' said Dan.

---

[1] http://gutenberg.readingroo.ms/5/5/556/556-h/556-h.htm#link2H_4_0022

'Mean!' Pharaoh cried. 'Why it's what you—what we—it's the Sachems' way of sprinkling the sacred corn-meal in front of—oh! it's a piece of Indian compliment really, and it signifies that you are a very big chief.

I was not only struck by the significance of the value of cornmeal for ancient people, but also its usage to show honor to the gods, as well as to the Great. So is it surprising that when the first pilgrims came to North America, the Native Americans taught them how to grow corn, because it was on this precious grain that they would survive and build their colonies.

So naturally corn bread and corn cakes were made with corn grown on the fields. 2 ½ acres of corn fed a family of three in the mountainous regions. In the plains, where the soil was richer, more people could be fed on lesser land, but richer and much better irrigated.

Any leftover corn apart from the bit which would be kept as seed corn for harvesting the next planting season was strictly for the chickens and for the hogs.

A standard cornpone recipe is made up of – **1 cup cornmeal, 1 teaspoon salt, ¾ cup boiling water, 1 tablespoon lard or fat.**

Combine the meal and the salt and while blending, gradually add water. Melt the fat in the baking pan. After the pan is greased, poured the surplus back to the mixture and blend well.

The mix should not more than 1 inch thick in the baking pan to start with – it will rise very little. If you want to make it rise like cornbread, you can add 2 teaspoons of baking powder. The cornpone will develop a rich brown crunchy crust. 50 to 60 minutes baked in a 350° oven is going to get you fresh, delicious home-baked cornpone

In olden days, it was usually baked in a step oven on the wood stove, or it was fried on a griddle, where a stove lid was removed. This cornpone and cornbread was the staple diet in the mountaineer diet in the USA for more than hundred fifty years. With greens, called "salit greens," meat and cold milk, this was good eating all around the year.

So how did grandma prepare salads?

In her days, salads were served as part of the meal, but nowadays, they are served as appetizers as accompaniments to the main course, or as separate courses following or preceding the main course.

When chicken, seafood and cheese are included, a salad plate is a good main course. You can also serve fruit salads as dessert.

Corn Cakes

This was normally fried on a griddle. These cakes were traditionally served with butter and eaten as a bread or they were served with sorghum molasses, and there you are, instant pancakes. Try them for breakfast.

One egg, beaten slightly, 1 cup cornmeal, half cup flour, 1 teaspoon salt, 1 cup hot water or milk, 1 tablespoon fat or lard, 1 teaspoon sugar.

Mix all the dry ingredients together. Then stir in all the others. Drop or pour on a hot and greased griddle surface. Fry until the cakes are golden brown on both sides. Serve with syrup or with butter.

Vegetables

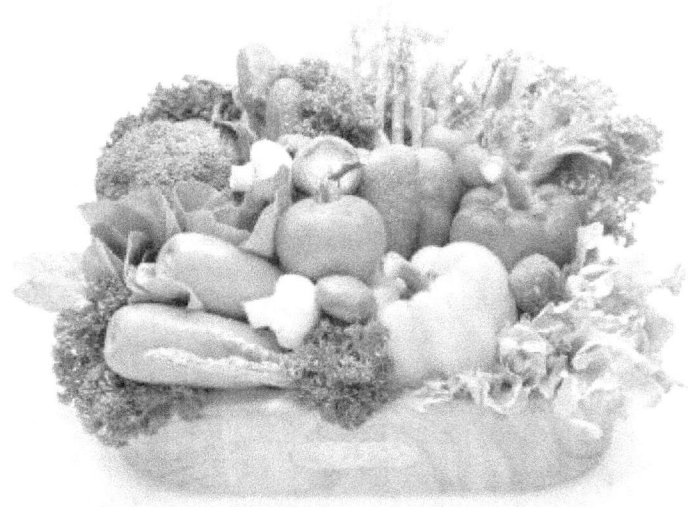

Two servings of Green, leafy and fresh vegetables should at least be served every day. You can cook yellow and green vegetables to get the vitamin A content and raw vegetables can be made into salads. Potatoes, which are relatively inexpensive and are available all throughout the year are going to supply you with vitamins and minerals.

Choose a variety of vegetables because they all differ in appearance, taste, cost and food values, when you are making up your meals.

Choose green and yellow vegetables frequently and those that can be served raw.

Choose canned or frozen vegetables only when you do not have fresh produce around. Choose these vegetables for brightness of color, freedom from blemishes, discoloration and soft spots. Learn to recognize the appearance of freshness and good quality.

Choose only the quantity of fresh vegetables that can be stored properly and used when the quality is still high.

How to Store Vegetables

Store the fresh vegetables for as short a time as possible in a cool, moist, and dark place. An exception is onions, which are going to keep better in dry storage. I normally keep my choice of onions in a basket right on top of the kitchen counter, tucked away in a corner. This gives me easy access to these onions whenever I need to chop, slice and dice them.

Wash the salad vegetables, trim, if necessary, drain and store in a vegetable crisper or in plastic bags in the refrigerator.

Leave fresh corn in the husks and peas in the pod and store in refrigerator until you need them.

Remove the tops of the beets and carrots, wash and trim and store in a cool place. Fresh beet tops can be cooked, just like spinach and are about as nutritious.

Frozen vegetables, if used, should be put into the freezer as quickly as possible after you purchase them. You may cook them without pre-thawing- an exception is corn on the cob, which has to be thawed first, otherwise you are going to get a soggy mess.

When you are storing food away properly, including vegetables and place items in the freezer, could the expire ration date on the package, so you know how old it is. Some items have a tendency to get lost in the freezer and then are taste less or have freezer burn.

Meat products can be frozen for up to six months, before the test and quality starts going bad.

Items such as apples and lettuce are going to go bad quickly, if you store them with brown spots. So remove those bad apples. Otherwise they are going to spoil the rest of your stored vegetables. And this is the truth, not a cliché or an idiom.

Preparing Vegetables for Cooking

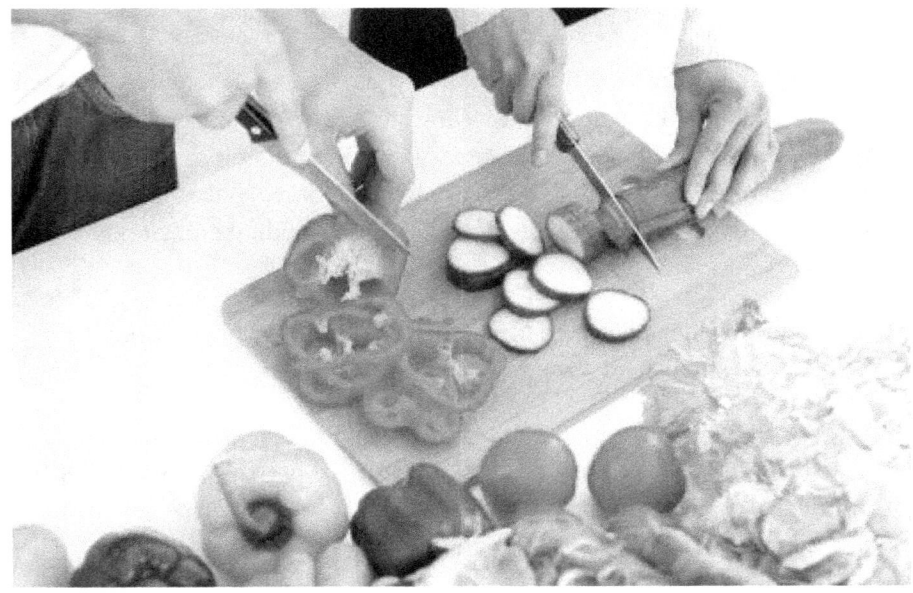

Preparation of the vegetables for cooking is going to depend upon the variety, the method and with individual customs and preferences. Whatever the method, the vegetables should be peeled as thinly as possible, or scrubbed until they are thoroughly clean.

Now you may say that the peel has plenty of nutritional value, so why am I advising you to peel it? That is because in many cases, these vegetables have been dusted with chemical pesticides. Those pesticides may have accumulated in the peel. So get rid of the peel. However, if you have grown these vegetables right at home, and have been using organic pesticides, you can keep the peels on, especially for potatoes, which can then be baked in their "jackets".

You can either leave the vegetables, whole or cut them into fairly large pieces to preserve their food values. Cook only enough for one meal to save the nutritional value and flavor.

Cook only until they are just tender. Overcooking is going to reduce the nutritional content, destroys the color and flavor and is often responsible for turning people against vegetables.

When boiling vegetables, add these prepared vegetables to a small amount of vigorously boiling water – half to 1 inch deep. Cover tightly. When the water returns to the boil, reduce heat to keep the water boiling gently.

Potatoes and beets require a little more water. Leafy green vegetables will cook over moderate heat in the water, which clings to the washed leaves. In fact, I cook spinach for storage just by washing it well and putting it in a cooker with just a teaspoon of salt and a couple of teaspoons of water, so that it does not burn. Two minutes later, the spinach is ready for cooling, grinding and storing away in the freezer.

Whenever I need some spinach, I just take out the quantity I need from the already parboiled spinach, allow it to defrost and cook it. Fast to cook, good to eat.

The color of the green vegetables may be better is the plan is uncovered for two or three minutes at the beginning. I found that adding a little bit of salt also preserves the color, especially when I am boiling peas

Cook until just tender. Drain and use the liquid in any gravy or sauce you are preparing. Season to taste, add butter if desired, and serve at once. You can use these boiled vegetables for salads too.

Steaming Vegetables/Meat

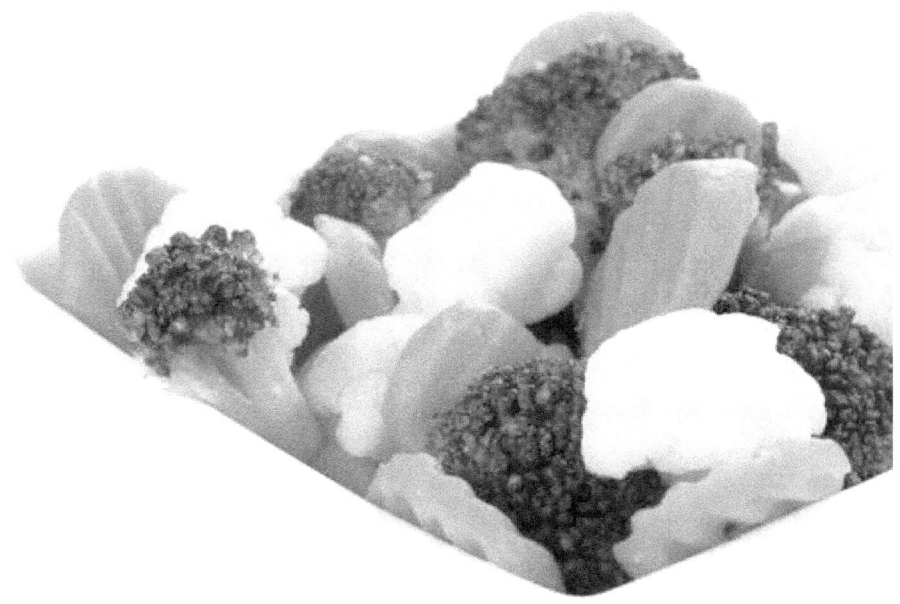

Steaming vegetables not only keeps the shape and texture, but it also retains the color and flavor of the bite sized pieces.

This method is going to take longer than boiling, but it retains the flavor and appearance. Place the prepared vegetables in a perforated section of a steamer, over boiling water, cover and cook until just tender. Season and serve at once.

This is a good method of cooking the vegetables, forest, you. The meat is going to simmer in the lower section of the steamer and the prepared vegetables can cook in the perforated section. So you save on electricity and time.

Now here is another tip. My father found it sad that he would not eat juicy pieces of meat because of the paucity of teeth and his dentures did not allow him to bite into meat which had not been overcooked into a mush.

Boiling the meat beforehand before cooking it just made it stringier, especially pieces of pork. It also got rid of the flavor, even though the soup water made the gravy tastier. I soon found out that steaming meat makes it soft and so palatable, that now he can enjoy juicy pieces, fatty pieces, and even pieces with the gristle, if they have been steamed beforehand.

So if you have an elder in the family who is missing out on juicy meat because of difficulty in chewing, steam the meat beforehand. Then cook it, bake it, broil it, sheesh kebab it or do what you will with it. This pre-steamed meat is going to be as soft as butter and does not lose out on texture and shape.

Cooking Frozen Vegetables

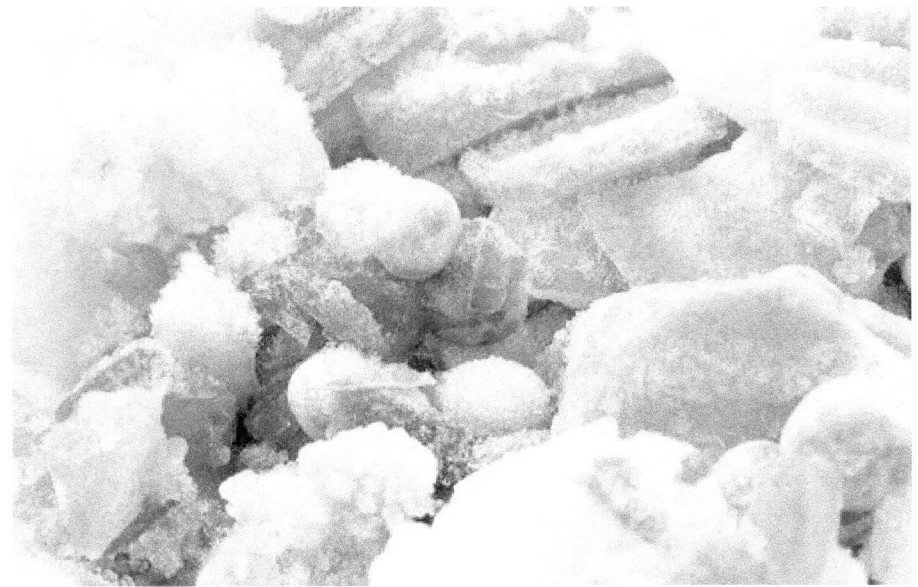

If you are using frozen vegetables, add them [except corn on the cob] to a small amount of boiling water over high heat. Break up the block with a fork, as it begins to thaw.

When the water returns to the boil, reduce the heat and boil gently until just tender.

Frozen vegetables require less cooking than fresh ones – from ½ to 2/3 of the time.

Suitable frozen vegetables may be sealed in an aluminum file or placed in a tightly covered casserole with butter and seasonings. You can then bake them in a moderate oven until they are just tender. If they are foiled – wrapped, they may be cooked on an outdoor grill.

Cooking Canned Vegetables

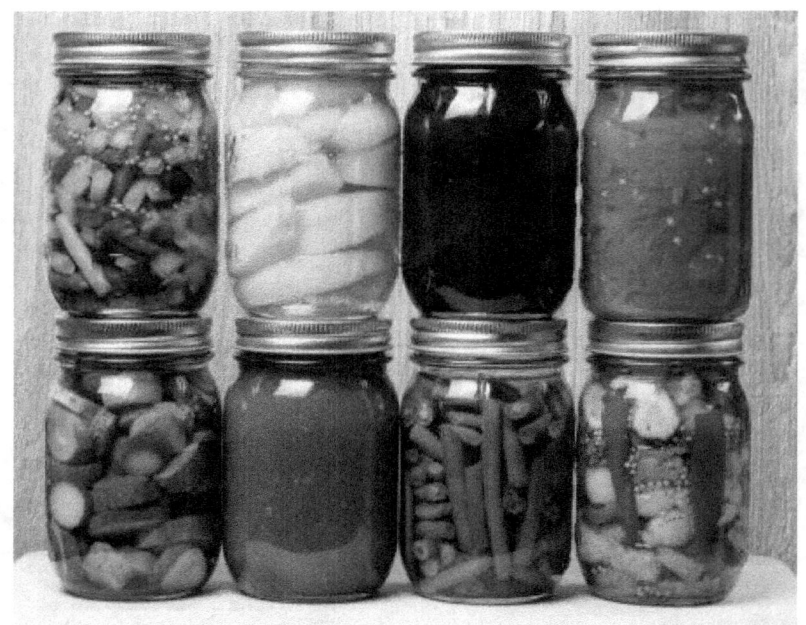

If the vegetables have been bottled, just use the amount you need, along with their preserving liquid.

Canned vegetables are already completely cooked and only need to be thoroughly heated for serving. Pour the liquid from the can into a saucepan and heat until boiling. Add the vegetables and leave over moderate heat until heated thoroughly. Season and serve at once.

Any remaining liquid is going to add flavor to sauces, gravy and soups.

How to Prepare Salads

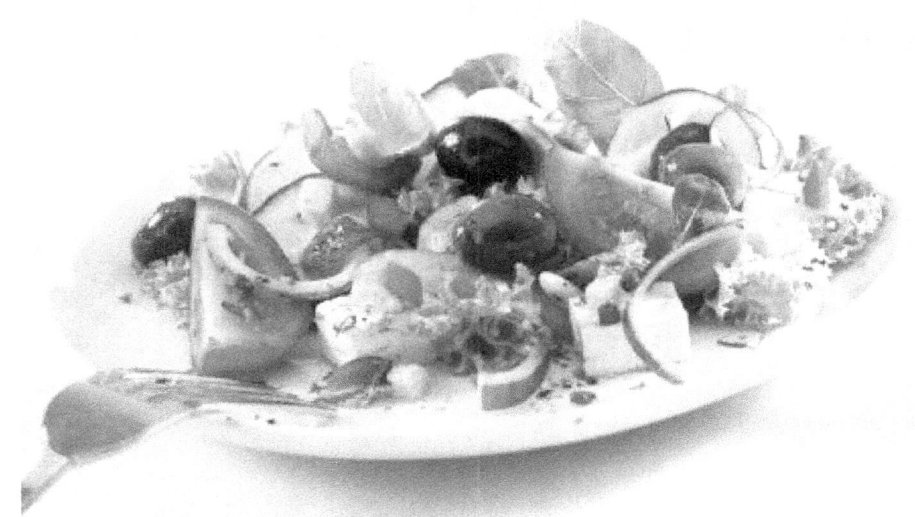

Pick up fresh salad greens, washed thoroughly in cold water. Drain well and store in the refrigerator – in vegetable crisper or plastic bags.

Wash other fresh vegetables and chill all the other ingredients including salad dressing before making a salad.

The Salit [salad] should be mixed, just before serving, although many of the ingredients may be prepared ahead of time.

Use a sharp knife to cut the ingredients of the salad. Choose a variety of shapes – slices, cubes, fingers, rings and slices, but have the pieces large enough to retain their character before and during mixing.

Chill the salad bowl and serve in chilled plates or bowls.

Add the dressing, just before serving, unless the recipe indicates otherwise. Use only just enough of dressing to coat the ingredients and combine by tossing the mixture lightly with spoon and fork.

Taste, adjust and add your seasonings if necessary.

Arrange attractively in serving bowl or in individual bowls or in salad platter or plate.

Suitable garnishes can include one or more of the salad ingredients in a different form. Here are a few simple examples –

Sprigs of fresh parsley, watercress, mint or tops of celery

Red pepper, green pepper strips, celery, cucumber and carrot.

Slices of tomato, cucumber, onion, radish, lemon and hard cooked egg.

Curls of celery, carrot, or raw turnip.

Ripe or green olives, pickles, radish roses, green onions.

Salad greens.

Tossed Salads

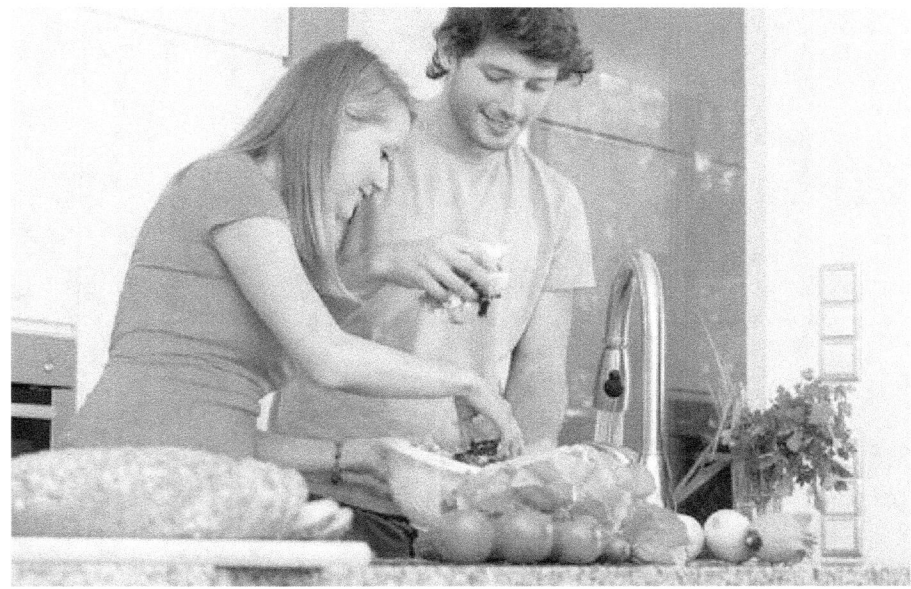

A healthy salad can be made by using any ingredient like green vegetables and leftover meat pieces

Start with crisp salad greens, cut or break into bite size pieces and place into the bowl. Add other vegetables as desired. Just before serving, add just enough dressing to coat the ingredients and toss lightly.

A simple tossed salad is going to consist of torn leaf lettuce or head lettuce and mild onion rings.

Other vegetables may include diced celery, sliced radish, strips of green or sweet red pepper, slivered carrots, grated turnip, chopped green onions, sliced cucumbers, sections of tomatoes or halved cherry tomatoes.

Cole Slaw

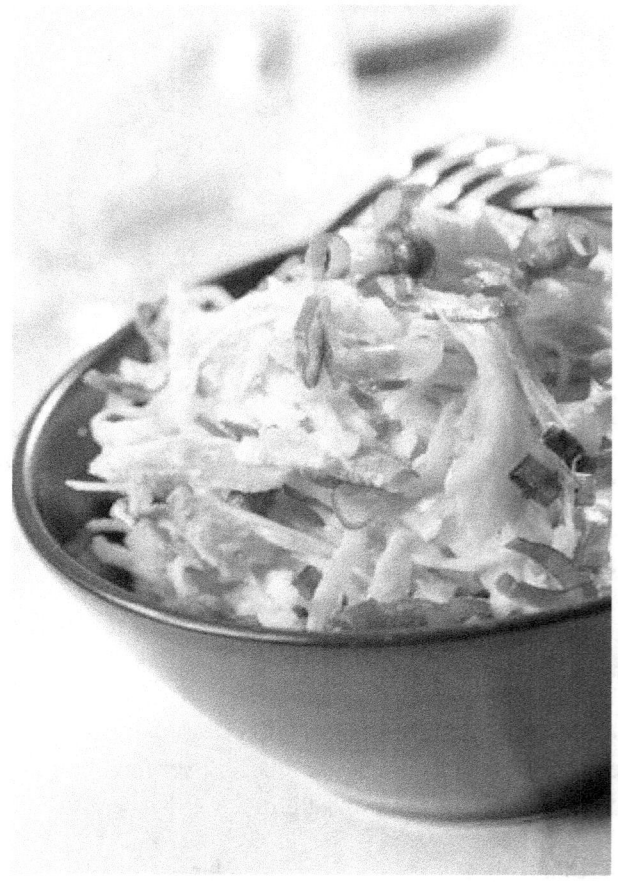

The traditional coleslaw is made in this manner –

1 cup sugar, 2 tablespoons mayonnaise, ¼ teaspoon salt, few grains pepper, 2 tablespoons melted butter, one egg, ¾ cup light cream, 1/4 cup vinegar, pinch of paprika, 4 cups shredded cabbage.

Combine the sugar, mayonnaise, salt and the part stop between the egg. Add melted butter and cream. Mix well.

Add the vinegar, very slowly while cooking over hot water, stirring all the while, until the mixture thickens. Chill.

Toss the dressing with shredded cabbage. Sprinkle with paprika.

Nowadays, this version of cottage cheese coleslaw, without the cream and mayonnaise is much appreciated by weight and health conscious people who have plenty of green vegetables around. Or you may just try it out as an unusual and healthy salad.

 This is going to be made with these basic ingredients – **6 cups cabbage, shredded, half teaspoon salt, few grains of pepper, and cooked salad dressing or sour cream dressing, half a teaspoon of caraway seeds.**

After that, you can add these items according to availability. **1 cup diced apples, and half a cup of seedless raisins. 1 cup shredded carrots and ¼ cup chopped nuts. 1 cup diced or sliced celery and want these phone finely chopped onions, some strips of green pepper or pimento is going to give color, 1 cup shredded red cabbage and ¼ cups of sweet/dill pickle.**

Now get together half a cup of cottage cheese, half a cup of mayonnaise, 3 tablespoons of vinegar, one onion.

Combine the cottage cheese and mayonnaise. Add the vinegar, and onions seasonings and caraway seeds. Combine the dressing with cabbage, apples, and green pepper and all the other items, you collected according to availability.

Place in large bowl lined with cabbage leaves. Garnish with cottage cheese and green pepper.

Serve chilled. This makes 8 to 10 servings.

Coleslaw Dressing

1 pint salad dressing, half a cup of vinegar, half a cup of cream or evaporated milk half a cup of sugar, one teaspoon celery seeds, one teaspoon salt, 1 ½ tablespoons prepared mustard, a little bit of garlic salt, dash of pepper.

Blend all the ingredients sensual. Serve over chopped or shredded cabbage. Pour over just before serving.

What Is Salad Dressing?

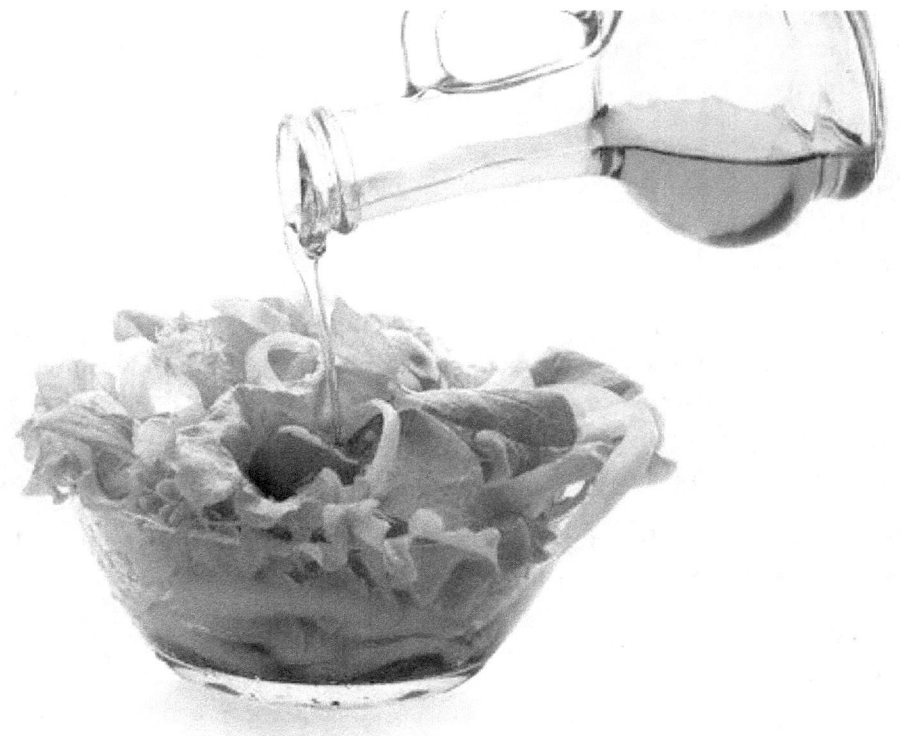

This is normally a mixture of vinegar and oil along with a number of herbs and flavorings, added to salads. Olive oil is best for salad dressing.

Potato Salad

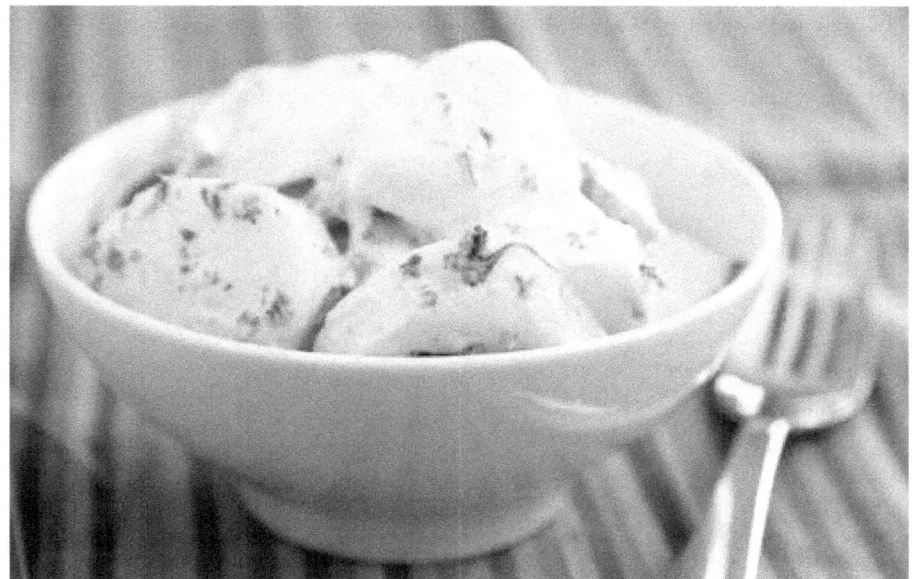

This was made very often, whenever grandpa had a bumper potato crop. In fact, grandma served these potatoes as often as she could.

4 cups cooked and diced potatoes, 3 tablespoons chopped sweet or dill pickles, ¼ cup cooked salad dressing, ¼ cup diced onions, 1/4 teaspoon celery salt, 1/tablespoons paprika, one teaspoonful salt.

Combine the potatoes and pickles in a bowl. Stir into the salad dressing, the diced onion, celery salt, paprika and salt. Combine with potatoes and pickles. Chill. Serve six.

Potato Salad Dressing

Beat **three eggs with half a sugar and half a cup of vinegar. Add 2 tablespoons butter, 1 teaspoon dry mustard, half teaspoon salt to taste, pepper.** Cook in double boiler or over low heat, stirring until thickened. Pour over potato salad.

Traditional Mayonnaise

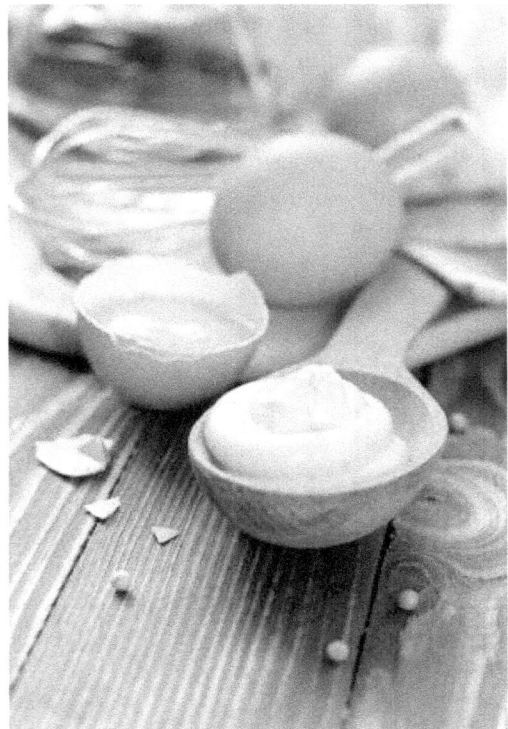

Mayonnaise is basically a French culinary creation, but there are plenty of delicious versions of mayonnaise adapted according to the ingredients available, all over the world.

Grandma's traditional mayonnaise was made up of **three eggs well beaten, to which half a cup of sugar and half a teaspoonful of mustard** was added. Then she added 1 **cup of cream, half a cup of vinegar,** adding the vinegar very slowly.

This mayonnaise was cooked in a double boiler until it was thick. Do not boil because that will spoil the cream.

Add half a teaspoonful of salt, when the mixture is cooled. You get 1 pint of delicious mayonnaise dressing with this recipe.

Conclusion

This book is full of tips and techniques on how to prepare food items and preserve them so that you can get full value for your dollars.

Along with old traditional recipes, you can get easy to utilize steps with which you can keep your food for a longer period of time in this book. You may want to look for more grandma cooking series books, giving you more tips and techniques, as well as recipes which have been passed down the ages and which often use very easily available ingredients.

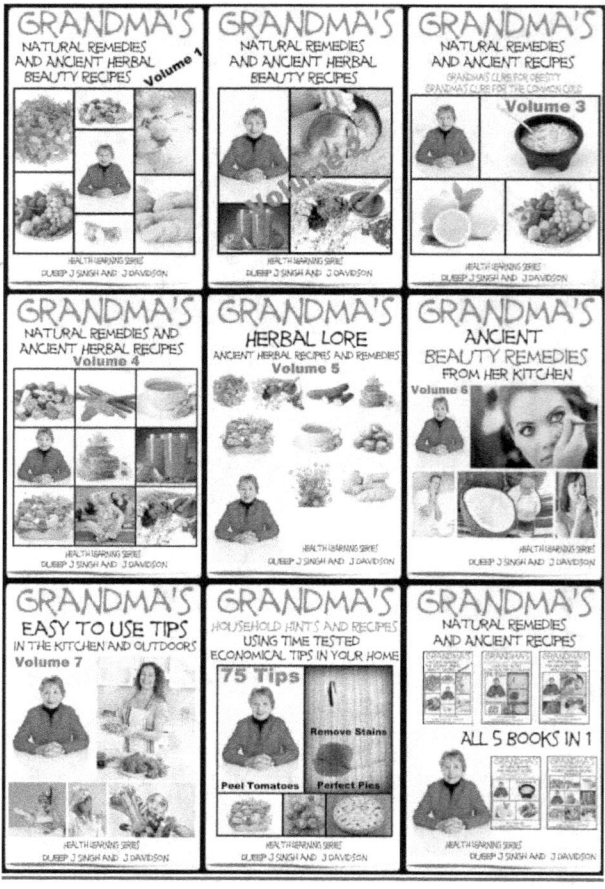

Live Long and Prosper!

Author Bio

Dueep Jyot Singh is a Management and IT Professional who managed to gather Postgraduate qualifications in Management and English and Degrees in Science, French and Education while pursuing different enjoyable career options like being an hospital administrator, IT,SEO and HRD Database Manager/ trainer, movie , radio and TV scriptwriter, theatre artiste and public speaker, lecturer in French, Marketing and Advertising, ex-Editor of Hearts On Fire (now known as Solstice) Books Missouri USA, advice columnist and cartoonist, publisher and Aviation School trainer, ex- moderator on Medico.in, banker, student councilor ,travelogue writer … among other things!

One fine morning, she decided that she had enough of killing herself by Degrees and went back to her first love -- writing. It's more enjoyable! She already has 48 published academic and 14 fiction- in- different- genre books under her belt.

When she is not designing websites or making Graphic design illustrations for clients , she is browsing through old bookshops hunting for treasures, of which she has an enviable collection – including R.L. Stevenson, O.Henry, Dornford Yates, Maurice Walsh, De Maupassant, Victor Hugo, Sapper, C.N. Williamson, "Bartimeus" and the crown of her collection- Dickens "The Old Curiosity Shop," and so on… Just call her "Renaissance Woman") - collecting herbal remedies, acting like Universal Helping Hand/Agony Aunt, or escaping to her dear mountains for a bit of exploring, collecting herbs and plants and trekking.

Check out some of the other JD-Biz Publishing books

Check out some of the other JD-Biz Publishing books

Gardening Series on Amazon

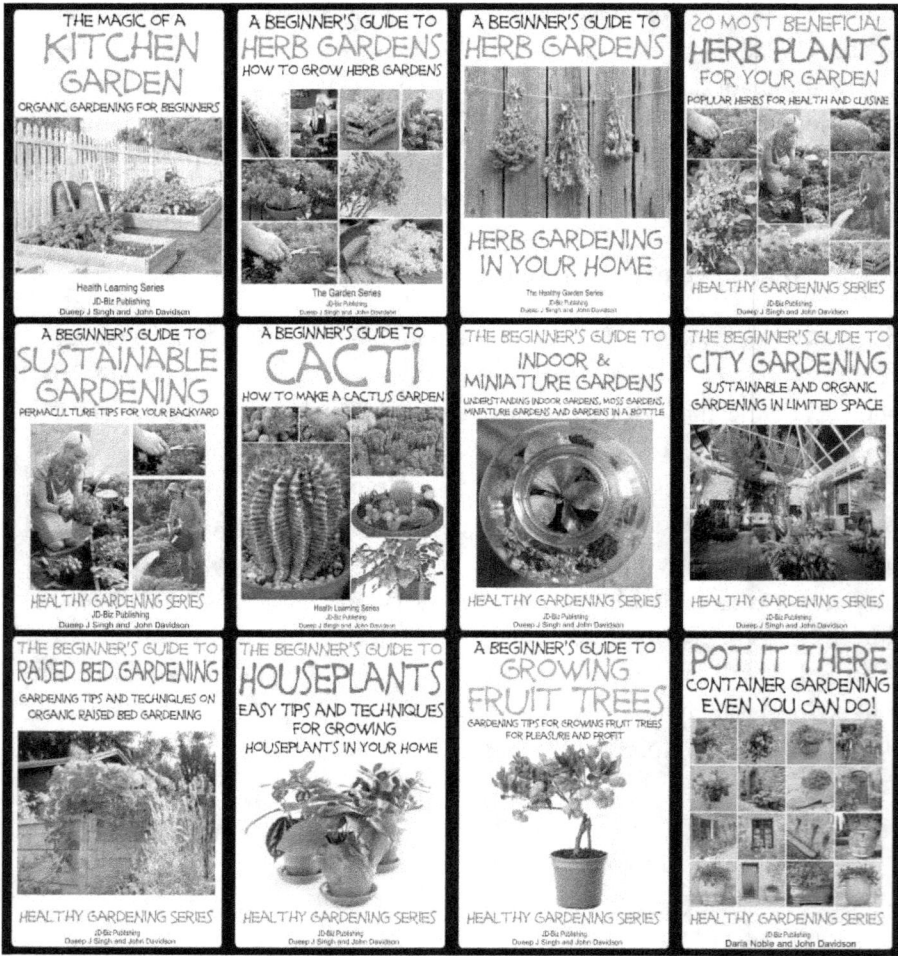

Health Learning Series

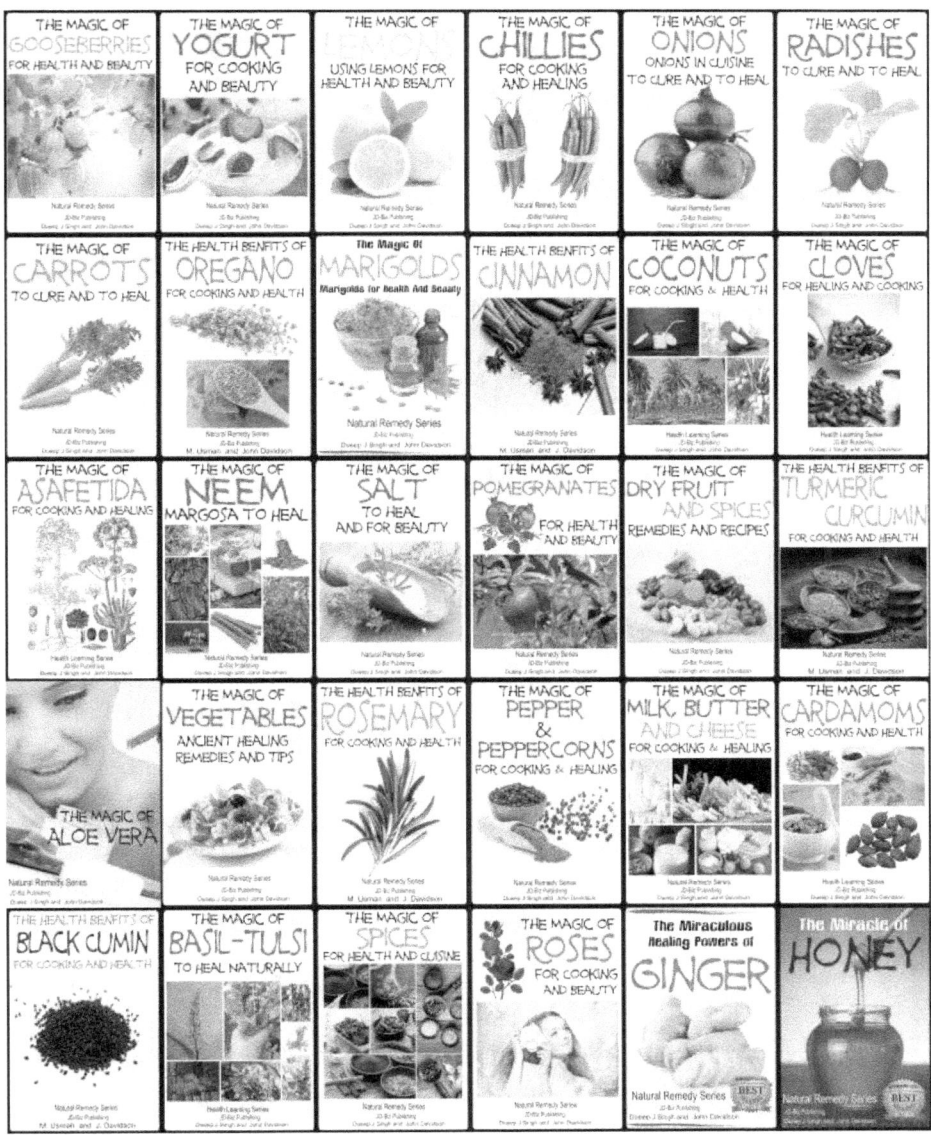

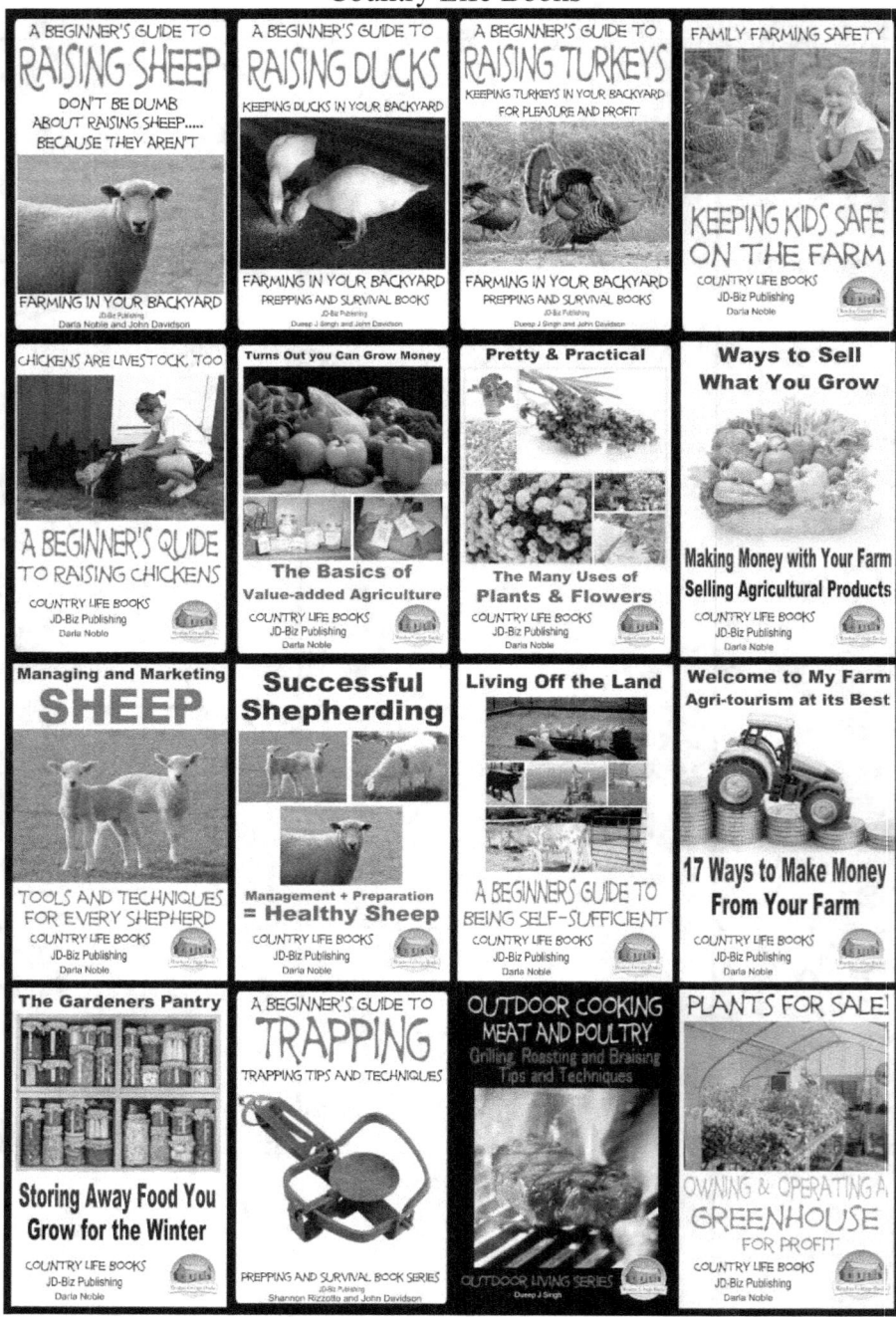

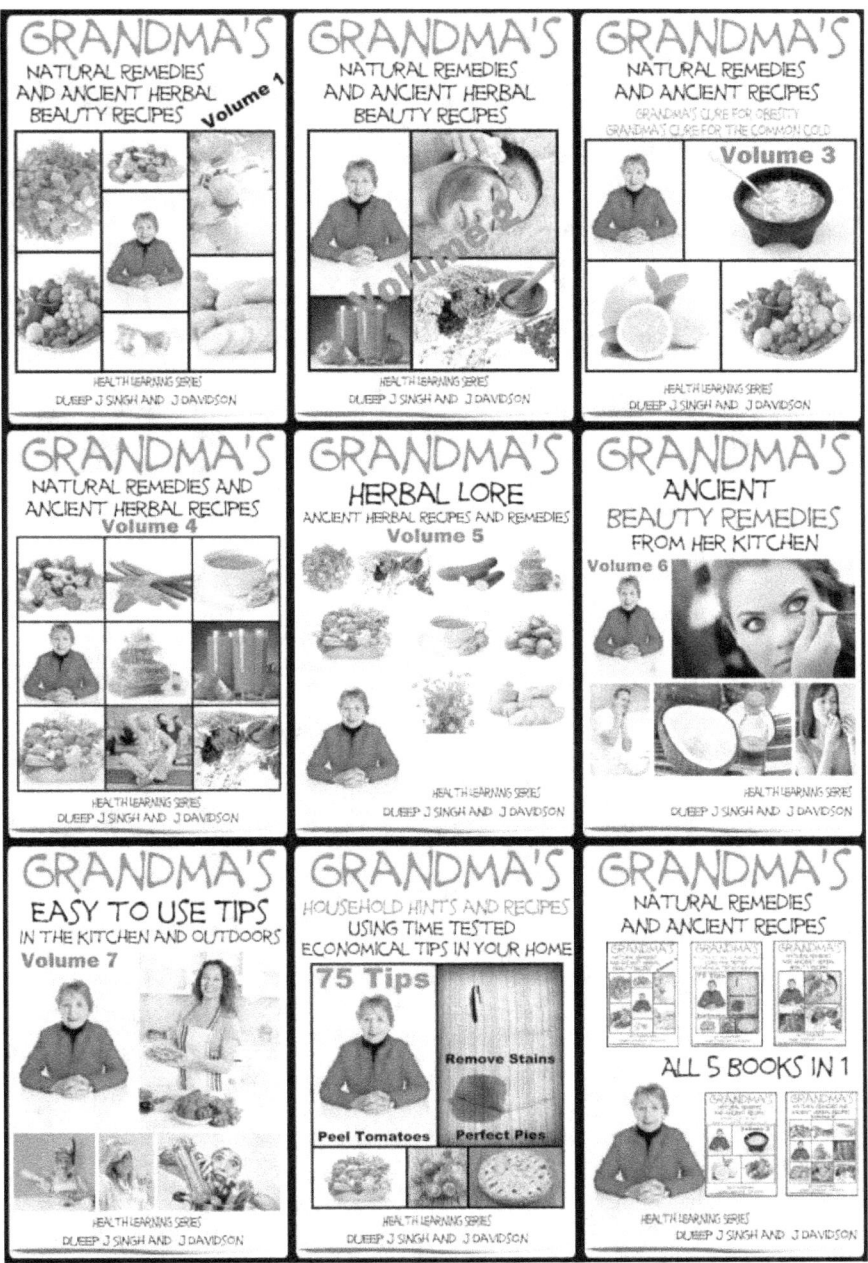

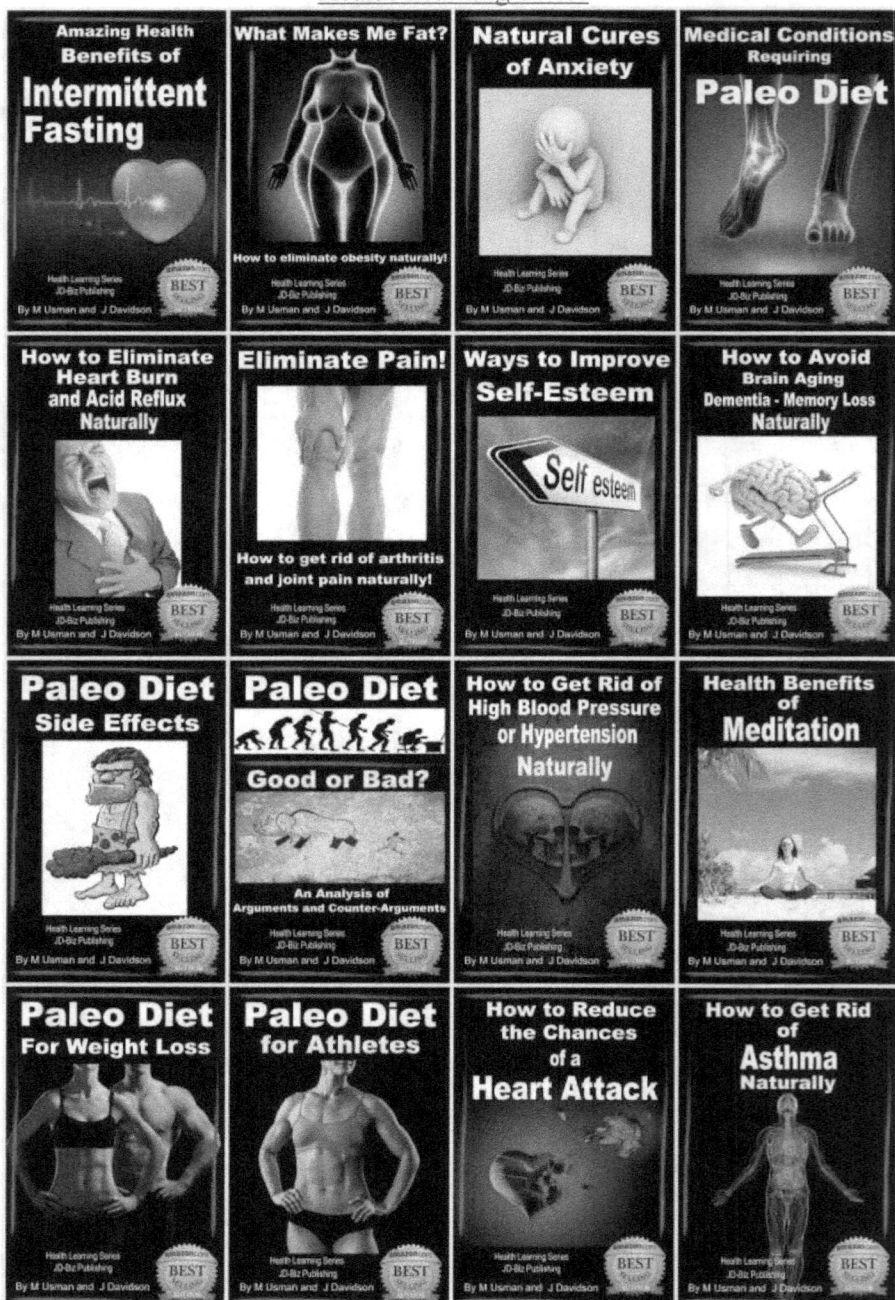

Amazing Animal Book Series

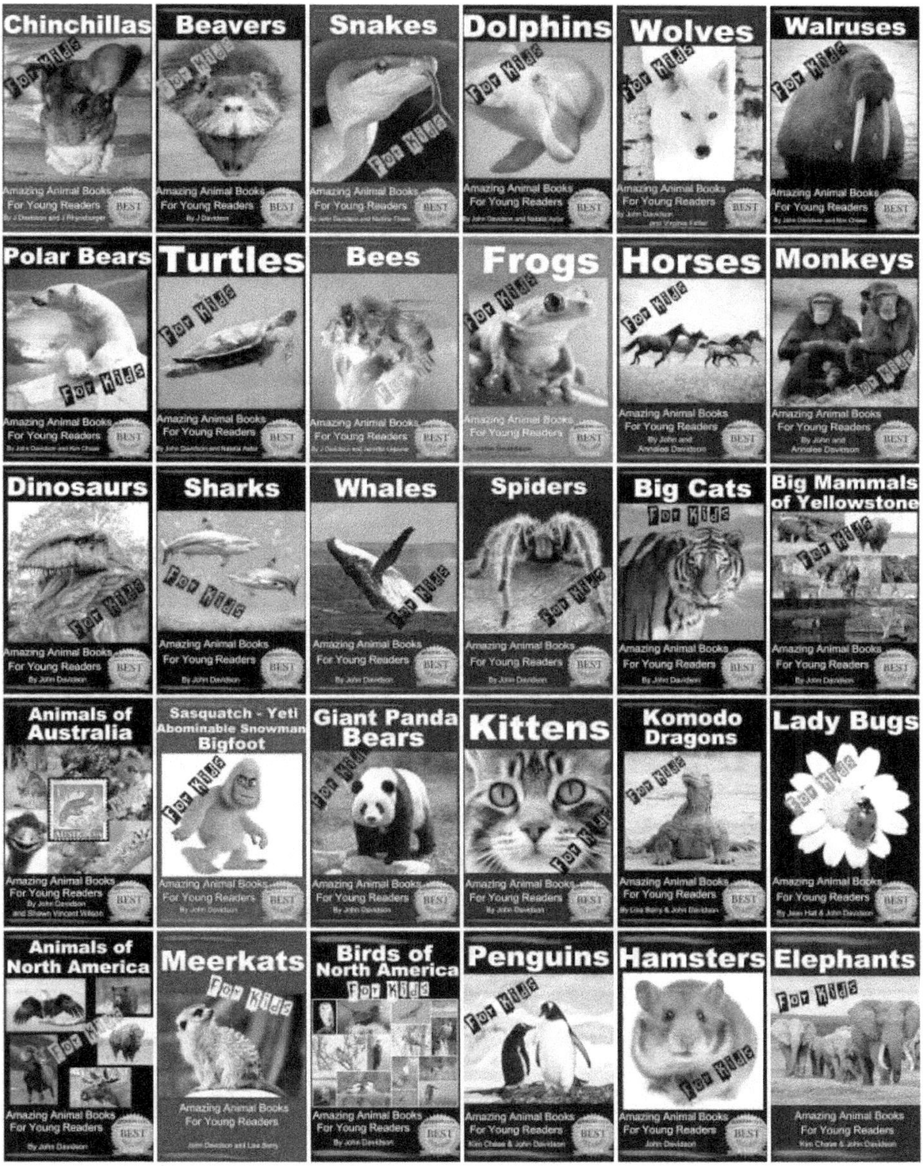

Learn To Draw Series

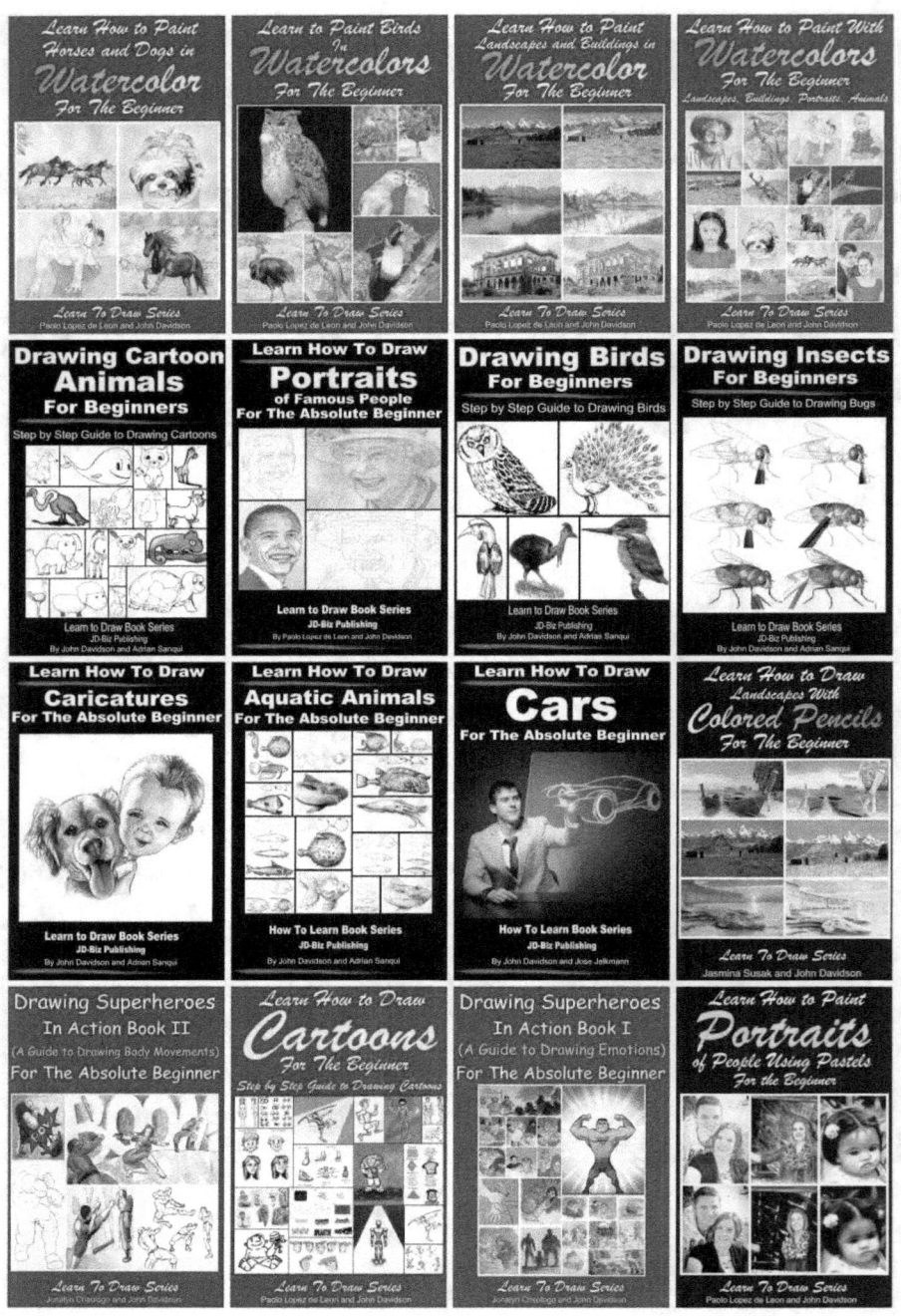

How to Build and Plan Books

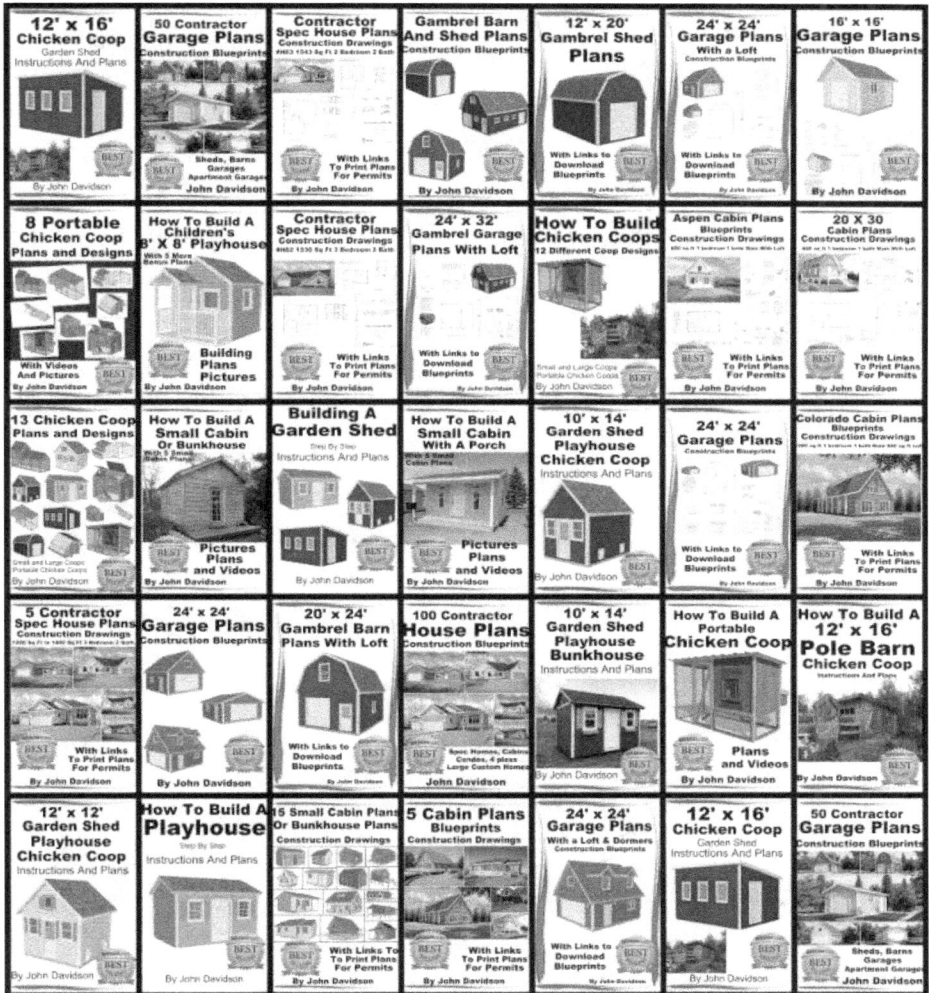

Entrepreneur Book Series

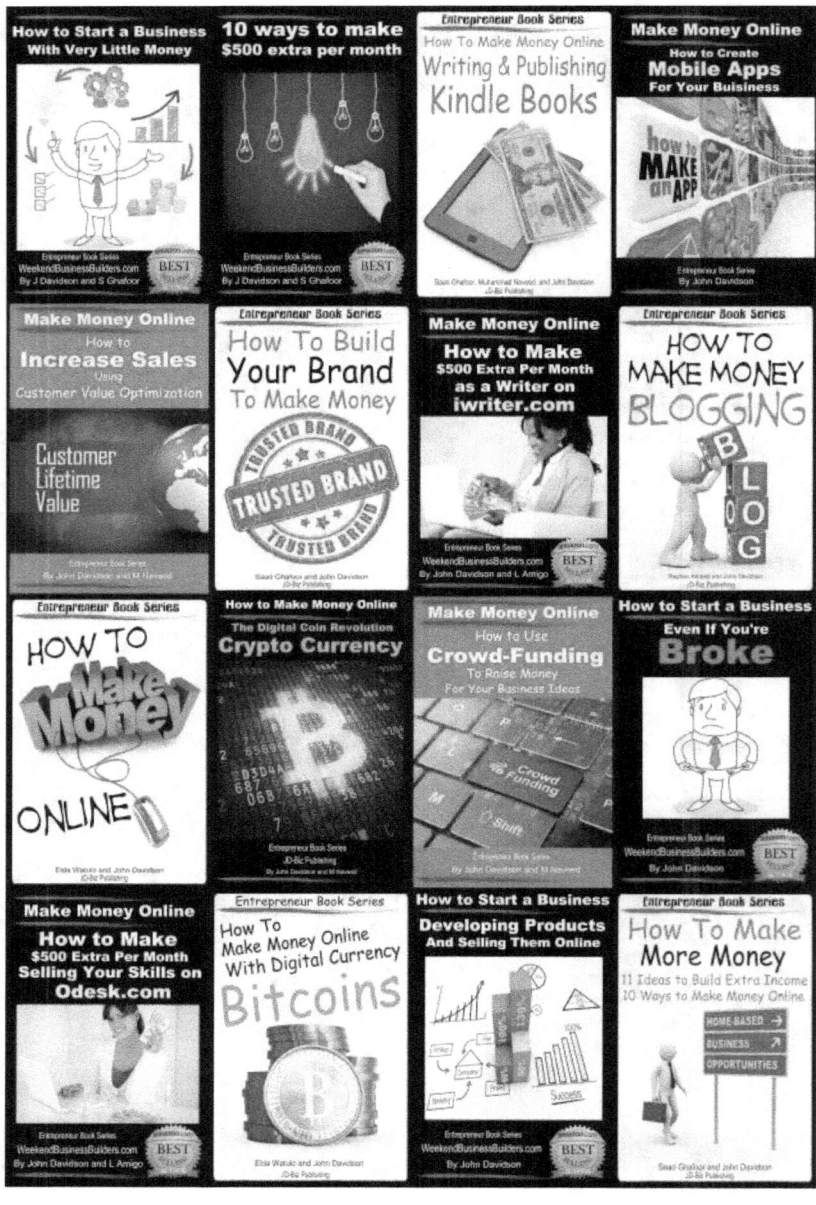

Our books are available at

1. Amazon.com

2. Barnes and Noble

3. Itunes

4. Kobo

5. Smashwords

6. Google Play Books

Publisher

JD-BIZ PUBLISHING

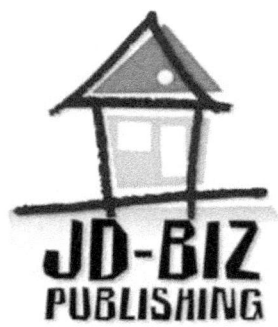

JD-Biz Corp

P O Box 374

Mendon, Utah 84325

http://www.jd-biz.com/

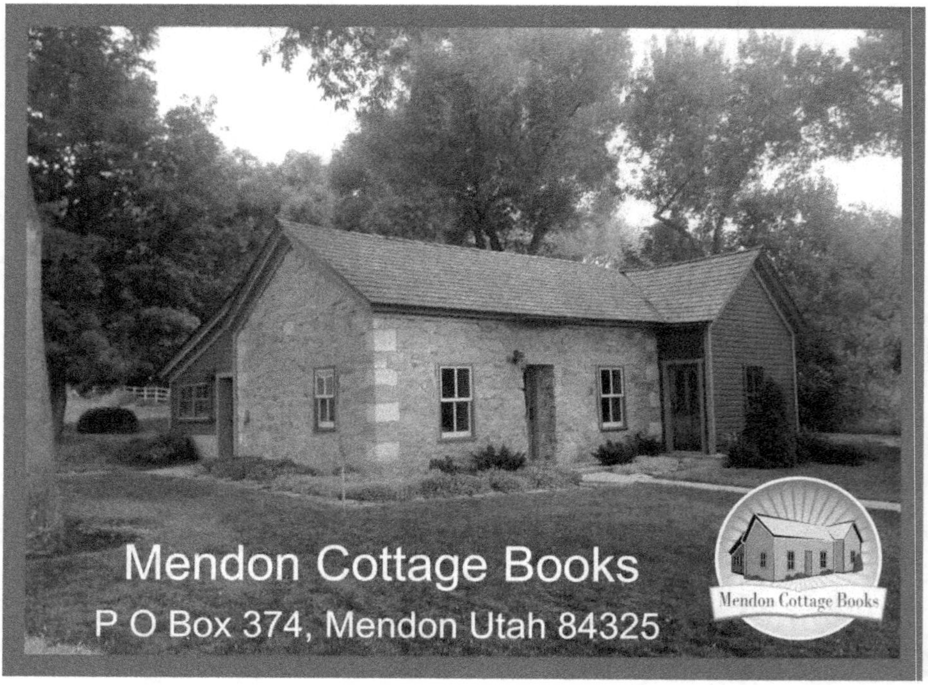

Mendon Cottage Books
P O Box 374, Mendon Utah 84325
Mendon Cottage Books

www.ingramcontent.com/pod-product-compliance
Lightning Source LLC
Chambersburg PA
CBHW071125280526
45787CB00003B/1167